The Gym Life
50 Ways To Improve Your Fitness

Take Your Training To The Next Level With Athlete-Tested Protocols For Building Elite Fitness

By Colin Stuckert
AGymLife.com

Contents

Tips Are Only Good If...

You Use Them!

It's going to be up to you to make your training, fitness and life *better through action*. I'm going to give you a bunch of ideas for what action to take but it'll still be up to you to take the action.

Upon reading the rest of this book, you now solemnly swear (or at least pinky promise) that you will get results by... Taking action!

Only through action comes result. You could read every fitness book, article, or forum in the world and ooze with more fitness knowledge than you can possibly contain, but how much result do you think you'll get if you don't put in the work?

This is what you'll get: ZERO. Zilch. Nada. No. None. Nane. A Google without a one in front of it. A billion x 0.

You are going to gain knowledge from what you are about to read, of that there is no doubt. But there is no guarantee that you will translate this knowledge into results.

"Knowledge is power only if applied." -Me

Yes, I just quoted myself. I've never heard this quote before so I'm trademarking it. It's mine. Next time you are trying to impress a date, you can use this quote as long as give me due credit: Just tell them to subscribe to my weekly newsletter at www.GymLifeClub.com to get a ton of free fitness, lifestyle and motivational related content!

No but really, I want you to read and act. The only way I am successful as an author is if you do that. Then, when you leave a review on Amazon (thank you, btw), it'll be easy to leave a positive one because you'll refer to the results you got from the action you took. You'll get results, be a happy camper and I'll have accomplished my mission of writing this in the first place. When this happens, we both win.

Let's both win... OK?

Good, I'm glad you agree. Now take out those black-rimmed spectacles you save for private use (or increase the text size on your Kindle) and let's get educating!

Yours in Fitness,

-Colin Stuckert

P.S. If you have any questions or comments, email me: ismynamecolin@gmail.com. I'm here to help.

50 Ways To Improve Your Fitness Training

1. Gear Up

My go-to gear includes: a pair of weightlifting shoes, two pairs of cross-training shoes (Reebok Nano's and Innov-8 195s), a speed rope, wrist wraps, boxing wraps, and comfortable and functional workout clothes. An investment in your gear is a worthwhile investment because it will make you more likely to do the work. Since you won't want to lose out on your investment (known as the sunk cost fallacy), you'll feel guilt if you don't use your gear to train.

Anytime you can guilt yourself into doing work, DO IT!

You can't buy results, but you can buy a higher likelihood you will get results by strategically investing in your food, supplements, and gear. These are worthwhile investments because they make your training easier and you more likely to stick with it.

2. Put On Your Shoes

Don't feel like training? Do this: put on your workout shoes and give it a few minutes. More often than not you'll find yourself headed to the gym.

Studies show that you are 70% more likely to go to the gym after putting on your workout shoes (or clothes). This simple act is the "trigger" that sets your subconscious in motion towards doing.

Use simple triggers like this to "trick" yourself into doing the work. Motivation isn't enough to keep you consistent all the time. You have to find ways to trick yourself out of motivational "ruts" that are a part of the results-getting process.

The hardest part of training when you don't feel like it is making the decision to go anyways. If you can *trick* yourself into working out, the rest is cakewalk. This is why triggers are so powerful. Essentially, you are tricking your subconscious into thinking you have made the decision to do something whether you really have or not. When you successfully tick yourself, the rest flows naturally.

Put on your workout shoes.

3. Time Your Warm-ups

Most trainees rush their warm-ups. They don't let their body get warm enough before moving to the more difficult parts of training. The term "warm-up" means to let your body rise in temperature. You want to do this your body needs to get closer to the higher body temperatures that will come during the workout. You don't want to go from "cold" to "hot" too fast as this can lead to injury and a reduction in performance.

The goal of your warm-ups should always be to move and break a sweat. The more you move, the more you get your body functioning at peak efficiency.

This is what I recommend: Set a stopwatch for 5 minutes and move. Incorporate some climbing, bodyweight exercises and dynamic stretching into your warm-ups. The more you move, the better. When the timer is up, you should have a sufficient sweat going. That is a warm-up.

4. Lift Heavy Weights

When I say "heavy," I mean heavy for you. Everyone's heavy is their own—it's relative to each individual. Always keep that in mind when you hear "heavy" as a recommendation.

Heavy is typically any weight over 70% of your 1RM (1 rep max). Constantly strive for training in this "heavy zone" and your total fitness will soar. (This goes for both men and women.)

5. Work Mobility Before And After Workouts

Your body is a complex machine of many moving parts. Just like a car, it becomes rusty and breaks down if you don't use it. The human body adheres to the "use it or lose it" rule.

To "use it" effectively, however, you can't just do random things and expect to target all of the many moving parts that make up the complex system that is your body. That would be like always changing the oil but sometimes forgetting to rotate your tires. You're just setting yourself up for problems.

You want to move your body in as many ways as possible. The more you move, the more you improve (that rhymed). Your body will have naturally weak areas, and you should spend more time on those. The only way you improve your weaknesses, or mobility in general, is to constantly work your weak areas.

Try incorporating Yoga, stretching and foam rolling into your program. They key to working mobility is to consistently utilize variety and making sure you are hitting as much as possible. Recommend resource: Becoming a Supple Leopard by Kelly Starrett

6. Get A Training Partner

You can also call your training partner your "accountability" partner because he or she is there to encourage you to show up and do the work. If you don't show up, you let them down. This is a powerful motivator for sticking with your program. Plus, you'll have someone there to spot you and keep you motivated.

7. Train On An Empty Stomach

This is known as training in the "fasted" state. Because digestion is so metabolically demanding, your energy levels are going to be greater when you train on an empty stomach. This might take some getting used to if you are used to eating before your workouts, but if you give it a week or two, you'll be astonished by the results (and you probably won't go back).

The handful of people I know that train in the fasted state all say the same thing: <u>They have more energy and drastically better workouts</u>.

8. Remember To Breathe

It's easy to forget to breathe when lifting weights. I tend to hold my breath more than I should during certain exercises (I'm working on it). You want to avoid this for many reasons, all of which help keep you safe. There are risks associated with training and holding your breath, notably increased pressure in your body. Furthermore, oxygen is integral to muscular performance, so if you aren't breathing, you aren't getting enough of it (duh).

Breathing for exercise: http://greatist.com/fitness/how-breathe-every-type-exercise

9. Steady Your Breath

Try to avoid big, gaping breaths that sap your energy and reduce your oxygen intake. Simply put, panting for breath is not a useful breathing strategy.

Focus on your breathing.

Try breathing in through your nose and out through your mouth at a steady pace. Your heart rate will steady when you focus and control your breath. This will give you control over your breath instead of it controlling you. Of course, this takes practice.

Always focus on your breath. Being aware of your breathing will allow you to control it... and the better you will perform as a result.

10. Show Up No Matter What

Let's say you aren't in the mood to train today (I'll play a violin for you). Here's what you do: put your shoes and workout clothes on, get in your car and turn it on. Then give it a minute.
9 times out of 10 you'll end up at the gym.

After you finish your workout, you should congratulate yourself because you took action instead of being a lazy sap (like most people).

Starting is the hardest part. Find "triggers" that get you started.

11. Don't Take Your Training Too Seriously

Give yourself a break. If you fail, get up and take solace in the fact that you are headed in the right direction. Without failure, resistance or setbacks, you can't improve. It's par for the course. It's the path to results land. It's absolutely necessary.

Seek failure. It's your path to better.

12. Use A Spotter And Go To FAILURE

If you aren't missing reps, you aren't training hard enough. Period.

13. Use Weaknesses To Warm-up

Focus on lots and lots of slow-to-medium reps during your warm-ups. I like to focus on my weakest movements during this time... so should you. If you struggle with the depth of your squat, hold the bottom while making subtle corrections to your form (knees out, active glutes) as you work through sets of 10. If you suck at push-ups, do super-solid reps with a slight pause at the bottom to rest and correct your form. Do then same thing other exercises.

Weaknesses are improved through repeating reps at a slow, deliberate, and form-conscious pace. This might seem like common sense, and it is, but most trainees don't put in the time.

One reason is because their Ego can't handle it. Spending time doing things we suck at, sucks. It makes us feel weak and incapable. Most of us like to train what we are good at because we like to feel strong. The thing is, training your strengths isn't the best use of your training time—training weaknesses is. Don't make this mistake.

Embrace your weaknesses. They are your path to improvement.

14. Practice Handstands Often

The best way (only way) to improve your handstand is to get upside a lot more than you do now. Obvious again? Ya, so why the hell aren't you getting upside down every day?

Here are a coupe ways to practice handstands:

- Kick up to a wall and hold for as long as you can.
- Do 5 kick ups (with plenty of room) and try to balance. Rest and repeat.
- Practice handstand walks.
- Practice negatives: Kick-up to a handstand on the wall and slowly lower your head to the ground.

15. Motivate Your Fellow Trainees

Offer a spot, a word of encouragement, and yell at them when they're struggling through a rep. This "gym karma" will always repay itself.

This is also a great way to make friends and build relationships. I've seen many great relationships start in the gym.

16. To Develop The Strict Pull-Up:

Have someone spot your ankles as you perform strict pull-ups. Push your ankles off their hands to assist reps and go to failure. This is the best way to develop the dead hang pull-up I have found. Get in as many reps and sets as you can.

17. Try Single Set Training

I'm a big fan of single-set training when it comes to the big lifts. There's nothing like an "all-out" set of squats to put your mind and body to the test.

Some coaches recommend only training with single-set training because they think it is the most effective method of eliciting muscular adaptation. I don't want to get into that here. Just know that this technique should be an integral tool in your training toolbox.

Jim Wendler's "5/3/1" program (which I thoroughly recommend) utilizes multiple warm-up sets that lead to a final "max rep" set. This is how I suggest you use single-set training in your program. Start with sets of 3-5 reps to warm-up incrementally as you get closer to the final max rep set. Your last set—the "all out" set—can be done at various percentages of your 1 rep max.

Let's look at an example:

Exercise: Back Squat
Starting Weight: 95 pounds
Last Max-Effort set: 205 pounds

Set 1: 135 for 3 reps
Set 2: 175 for 3 reps
Set 3: 190 for 3 reps

Set 4: 205 for max reps

As you can see, the warm-up sets use only a few reps and steadily increase in weight to get you closer to the last set. The last set is the "all out" failure set of as many reps as possible. Utilize a spotter on your last set so you can go to absolute failure.

Try incorporating single set training with some of the "big" lifts each week (squat, deadlift, press, bench). If you prefer it, you can use single set training for all of your big lifts, like I do.

18. Do A Max-effort Set of Push-Ups Every Morning After Waking

Your morning routine will prime you for the day ahead. What better way to start the day then with a nice "pump" and juicy influx of feel-good exercise hormones? (That was rhetorical... but possibly the answer is: "morning sex.")

19. Build A Morning Routine... And Stick To It

A common theme among fit (and successful) people is they usually have a morning routine that starts their day off with intention.

I've developed a routine naturally over the years, but it wasn't until the last year or so that I started to make a conscious effort to improve and refine it.

The most common components of a morning routine include exercise, a glass of water, coffee, supplements, meditation, writing, reading, stretching, and positive affirmations. Your routine will be your own. Try experimenting with each of these and see how they work for you.

This is my routine (I have a printed checklist in the bathroom I follow):

1. Wake up and immediately do 20 push-ups and pull-ups.
2. Bathroom affirmations in mirror (I have my list and I mix these up from time to time)
3. Glass of water + the following supplements: Ciltep, Cod Liver oil, Vitamin C, Vitamin D (if not getting sun)
4. Bulletproof Butter coffee (recipe here... it's amazing: http://agymlife.com/how-to-make-bulletproof-butter-coffee/)

5. Read 20-30 pages of whatever book I'm working through
6. Start work for the day

I might rearrange this order from time to time, but mostly this is what I do every morning. I'm currently working on adding a few minutes of mediation to this routine.

What does your morning routine look like?

20. Take Your Training Seriously

Always strive to improve your training: *Put in your best effort every time.* Never accept what you have. Always strive for more.

As Bruce Lee said, "Be happy but never satisfied."

You want to develop a mindset of *constant improvement*. Training isn't a final destination; it's a lifelong journey.

Your training—and your life—will be much easier if you make it your default mindset to constantly seek improvement. You'll also get the benefit of having this seep into other parts of your life like your relationships, work, school, etc.

When you make it your mindset to always seek better, your results will come from many angles in many parts of your life, not just fitness.

21. Do A Few Strict Pull-Ups Every Day

This is one of my favorite fitness tips of all time. Since pull-ups are a low-rep exercise for most of us (meaning most of us only need a few reps to get a favorable adaptation), it's easy to get a healthy stimulus for growth every day using minimal reps.

22. Do A Few One-Arm Push-Ups Every Day

See #21. The same applies.

23. Meditate 5 Minutes A Day

Meditation can improve your entire life. The benefits are too many to list here. What I will tell you about meditation is it isn't complicated or require fancy cushions, robes, or expensive programs. All you need is to do is count your breath and empty your mind and you can elicit amazing positive changes in your life.

Check out the Headspace meditation app (or look into free guided meditation resources).

24. Do 30 Squats And 30 Push-ups After Every Meal

This will improve digestion and reduce fat-gain. You'll be amazed by how you feel after doing this, especially those times you overeat and feel *stuffed*. The credit for this technique goes to the book The 4-Hour Body by Tim Ferris.

Tim recommends you do these exercises before and during your meal for greater effect. This is especially effective when eating out.

We all do our body a disservice when we eat out. When I eat out, I use this technique about 90% of the time. The hardest part is remembering to do it. If I forget to implement this technique when I'm eating not so great, I'm quickly reminded when my stomach starts making weird noises.

The next time you eat a meal and start feeling that sickly, "full" feeling, go to the bathroom and do 30 squats and 30 wall presses. You'll be amazed by how quickly you start feeling better.

25. Walk After Every Meal

There is a Chinese proverb goes like this: "After a meal, walk a hundred steps to live to be ninety-nine."

Well, that pretty much sums it up, no?

Walking benefits: http://www.marksdailyapple.com/17-reasons-to-walk-more-this-year/

26. Use Heat

The sauna, steam room, hot tub and hot showers can improve recovery. They are also good for training your resilience (and a great place to get some mediation in).

27. Throw Things

Humans have been throwing spears, javelins and rocks for thousands of years.

28. Practice L-sits And Frog Stands Often

Basic gymnastic skills are a great way to build strength and mobility without infringing on recovery. By practicing a bit here and there, you'll strengthen your stabilizer muscles and improve your coordination and balance without too much stress to your CNS (central nervous system).

Gymnastics is a perfect way to train when your body is still in recovery mode.

29. Take Rest Days

Warning: the following might blow your mind. Are you ready? Strap in...

You can't train every day!

Phew, that was a close one. I can still imagine the gaping, mouth-wide-open look on some of your faces.

Listen, it's time to set a few things straight. First, the physiological processes in your human body when you exercise involves a breaking down of muscle fibers, a weakening of your central nervous system and a depletion of glycogen (fuel) in your muscles. This is good; it's what you want to happen when you train. But here's the thing...

...this isn't the process that makes you stronger and fitter!

The process that repairs your body and makes you stronger, bigger and faster is called *supercompensation*.

Supercompensation happens when your body over-compensates to the breakdown that was the result of training. This process comes after your body has had a chance to recover to where it was originally before training. Then, your body makes itself stronger so that it will perform better the next time it performs the same physical activity. This process of recovery then added adaptation is what builds more muscle fibers, better cardiovascular performance, and a more functioning system that will perform better the next go round. In short, this is you getting fitter.

When you break your body down, it adapts by building a better body... but only if you give it time in the recovery state! Since supercompensation comes after the recovery period, if you fail to let your body fully recover, it won't be able to supercompensate by getting stronger and fitter. This is called "overtraining."

Overtraining comes in many forms and has a lot to do with an individual's genetics. The most common form of overtraining in the plateau.

Let's review:

1. Training is the physical breakdown process.

2. The rest and recovery period helps your body come back to where it was before you started the training process.

3. Finally, after your body has recovered, supercompensation grows your body beyond where it was at the onset of training. When this happens you are a fitter human being. If you fail to give your body time to rest through he recovery and supercompensation stages, you get overtraining.

The way to avoid overtraining is to spend more time on your nutrition, sleep, active recovery, and throttling your volume back as needed.

Your body is a delicate balance of many things. If you are stuck or if your gains have slowed drastically, it's time to take a hard look at your program and find where you could use more rest and/or less volume.

Most people should take two full rest days a week and a full rest week every 2-3 months. Listen to your body and test and tweak to find what gets you the best results. Above all, make sure you give your body time. It can take years to build a world-class physique.

Remember: Training is the breakdown and rest is the build-up.

30. Do Home Workouts If You Can't Make It To The Gym

The beautiful thing about functional training is it can be done anywhere. You can achieve a high level of fitness using only body-weight exercises and metabolic conditioning from home. Of course, you should utilize a fundamental strength program to amplify your results, but it's important to showcase how easy it is to get a workout in whether you have access to gym and equipment or not.

How To Create Workouts With Your Body

Below is a simple system for creating hundreds of workouts you can do without equipment. These workouts are perfect for traveling athletes and serve as an excellent starting point for beginners.

The 9-bodyweight movements:

Squat
Push-up
Sit-up
Burpee
Lunge
Sprint
Plank
Broad Jump, Box Jump
Handstands, Press, Walks, Holds

Basic Workout Template:

Pick Exercises
Pick Reps Per Movement
Pick Rounds or Total Reps Goal
Pick Format: AMRAP (as many as possible) or a total # of reps or rounds
Set stopwatch and go!

Example: 10 rounds of: 5 Push-ups, 5 Air Squats, 5 Sit-ups.

Complete 5 push-ups, 5 air squats and 5 sit-ups. Repeat this 9 more times with proper form as fast as possible. Your score is the time you finish (the faster the better). Write your time down so the next time you do this workout you can compare results.

In only 15 minutes a day (or less) you can progress towards elite fitness using just your body and the ground. That's pretty freaking awesome if you ask me.

31. Train Farmer Carries

Farmer carries are one of my favorite exercises. They are a great way to build not just functional body strength but mental strength as well. They develop your grip, traps, upper-back, abs and brain.

I like to walk fast and make turns and pivots around obstacles to get all of my stabilizer muscles working. You can use dumbbells, kettlebells, buckets of sand, or any heavy object with a handle. Set a distance and challenge yourself to complete as many revolutions as possible.

The key to farmer carries (and holds) is to grit your teeth and go as long as you can.

32. Incorporate Strongman Work Into Your Program

Have you ever seen the Strongman competitions on TV? Those are fun to watch. You may not realize this but many of the training methods Strongmen use can produce amazing gains in functional full-body strength for you and I.

Exercises include sled pulling/pushing, picking up stones or other awkward objects, throwing, deadlifting, and farmer carries.

Humans are made to carry heavy and awkward things. What do you do with a freshly killed wholly mammoth or buffalo? You drag it back to your tribe, which is probably miles away. How do you save an injured solider on the battlefield? You pick him up, put him over your shoulder and run to safety.

The problem with training *only in the gym* is you are likely to develop physical imbalances from training movement patterns that are too rigid or predictable. This is why I'm a big fan of strongman and primal-style training. These methods put you off-balance and in awkward positions, which develops more physically well rounded fitness.

Check out YouTube for exercise ideas and start incorporating Strongman-style exercises into your program. You'll be glad you did. (My favorites are sled work, tire flips, and farmer carries.)

33. Do Strict Dips And Negative Holds On Rings

I love gymnastic rings. If you don't have access to rings, you can buy a set on eBay or Amazon. You really should. The strength development from training on rings with even the most basic exercises is out of this world!

Dips and holds on rings should be a training staple in everyone's program. If you are new to fitness, you might have to work with a band as you build the stabilizer strength necessary to avoid the *wobble*.

First focus on slow, strict dips; most trainees do ring dips poorly. It's rare you see athletes hit full extension at the top and full depth at the bottom of the dip.

If you don't have a set of rings you can do regular dips, "support" holds, which is the top portion of a dip for a hold, and the static hold at the bottom of the dip. These are great strength builders that are overlooked by most athletes.

34. Turn Wrists out At The Bottom Of A Muscle-up

This will ensure you reach full extension of the elbows, lats, and shoulders. This is a common "no rep" for athletes performing the muscle-up. They fail to hit full extension at the bottom of the muscle-up (and often, pull-up) because it takes more strength to avoid losing grip while performing reps.

You should always aim to perfect your movement. It will make you better. Personally, I'd rather know my reps were done with proper form. But that's just me. Some athletes like to assuage their ego with faster times and shoddy movement.

(Don't be like that.)

The Pull-Up: A common fault of the pull-up is failing to come to the full hang at the bottom with elbows and lats fully extended. Let your body come to a full hang at the bottom of the pull-up—arms fully straight at the bottom. Bent elbows = no rep.

35. Do Shoulder Dislocates Every Workout

This is a great mobility exercise for your upper body. To start, grab a dowel or broomstick and grip it as wide as possible. Then slowly raise it over and behind your head until you touch your lower back. Slowly return it to the front. If that was too easy, move your grip in a bit to decrease the width. It will become more difficult each time you decrease the width of your grip.

Try to find the sweet spot where you feel the stretch but don't have to force it. In time, your flexibility will increase.

36. Get Your Family Involved In Fitness

Bring them to the gym on a guest pass. Ask them to help you in the kitchen and show them tips for cooking healthy food. Take them to the park and climb the playground. Take a walk and have a conversation.

Then encourage them to continue these habits on their own.

Healthy habits can save lives. But you can't lecture or force people or you'll lose them. They have to come around on their own. The best you can do is encourage and motivate them by sharing your journey with them as much as possible.

Share progress as you venture through your health and fitness journey. In time, if you keep it up, they'll start coming around. I've seen it happen time and time again.

Because you are dealing with your family, their initial inclination might be to resent your advice. You should pretty much expect this... then ignore it. Keep on keeping on.

After a while, you'll notice as they start becoming more interested. This usually happens when they start asking you questions. They'll lean in and listen a bit more than they used to. Just keep doing what you are doing without being to obvious of your intentions.

Given time, they will probably start telling you about things they did on their own, like the healthy salmon they found at the store or how they went for a run. When this happens, the change has started. They have opened up to the concept and it's up to you to do anything you can **to help them!**

Your family is the only family you got. You don't want to bury them because of dumb, totally preventable causes like poor lifestyle and nutrition habits.

Get them involved in your health and fitness. Share your tips, techniques and stories. Motivate and inspire. This process could take years, but it'll totally be worth it.

37. Have A Recovery Plan

When your muscles become "sore" from training, the protective layer covering them known as fascia can accumulate tears that bunch and adhere together. These are known as "adhesions" and they prevent your muscles from operating at peak efficiency. Use Myofascial release to apply pressure and "roll out" (as it's often called) these adhesions. Doing so will restore proper function and improve recovery time.

How to use a lacrosse ball or foam roller to perform myofascial release:

Place the lacrosse ball or a foam roller (or a pvc pipe) on the ground or a wall. Find areas of your body that are painful when you apply pressure and slowly work through the pain to release the adhesions.

Common areas to target include the hamstrings, glutes, calves, quads, and all areas of the back up to the neck. Search "Foam Rolling" on YouTube.

It's best to roll out a before and after exercise as well as multiple times throughout the day.

Benefits of myofascial release:

Helps prevent injuries
Increases blood flow
Reduces soreness
Increases flexibility
Reduces tightness and knots
Speeds up recovery

Another recovery technique you can utilize is the "contrast shower." This is the switching of hot and cold water for intervals. Try 60 seconds hot and 30-45 seconds cold for 5 sets.

Stretching is another recovery technique you should be using often. This can vary between static, PNF, and active stretching. Check out YouTube for exercise demonstrations. A common mistake most people make with stretching is they don't spend enough time in their stretches. According to Kelly Starrett, author of "Becoming a Supple Leopard," the "minimum therapeutic dose" is two minutes. Meaning, it takes at least two minutes to get the full benefit from a stretch.

38. Hit Every Major Lift At Least Once A Week

These include: Squat, Deadlift, Press, Bench, Snatch, Clean, Jerk.

Many people get lost in the sea of possibility when it comes to training and fitness. **And it is sooooo unnecessary.** You ever wonder how the guys in prison are always so strong? They usually have access to only a bench and some dumbbells, if that. Yet they get crazy strong. This is because they stick to the basics <u>and they do a ton of freaking reps</u>. By being confined by what they don't have and can't do, they end up training a few movements using lots of volume. This is known as linear progression.

This is exactly what you should do to get gains.

The more you spread out your weight training (any training, really), the more you fail to target the linear progression that is necessary for massive results. To get big results, you have to stack your gains on top of each other by focusing on less movement and more volume. For example, if you want to improve your squat, it's best to squat consistently while increasing weight and volume as your body becomes stronger. The majority of your results will come from more squatting and not doing every leg exercise you can think of.

The point here is, if you are interested in building muscle and strength, you should be focusing on developing a short list of exercises and training them in a linear way.

Don't complicate weight training. Focus on the big lifts and do them consistently. Then train whatever else you want in between.

If you could only do 1 or 2 exercises for the rest of your life, what would you pick? The correct answer is: Squat or deadlift. No other exercise even comes close.

Recommend strength programs: 5/3/1 and Starting Strength

39. Do 10 Pistols Per Leg Every Day

Pistols are a great exercise that most of us struggle with. Most people can't do one pistol, let alone ten. As a result, doing a few reps every day can provide adaptation for most people (like strict pull-ups). Start training them every day.

If you are just starting out with pistols, and if you struggle with reaching full depth, use a chair, doorway or pole to assist you out of the bottom. Make sure your heel stays flat and your butt touches the back of your ankle in the full-seated position at the bottom. Work this movement slowly until you reach perfection.

40. Learn To Bounce Out Of The Bottom Of A Squat

If you struggle with the squat "rebound" that is part of a fluid squat, you should training lots of reps with a dowel before moving to an empty barbell. Lots and lots of reps is the key here (as is true of all weakness training).

By developing a fluid squat rebound, you'll be able to lift more weight. More weight translates to more development. (Seeing the trend?)

41. Always Be Learning

Fitness, nutrition, lifestyle, and the plethora of variables that go into this amazing thing called your body all require constant learning with an open mind.

Here are some of my favorite resources: www.GymLifeBooks.com, www.MarksDailyApple.com, www.GymLifeClub.com

42. Practice Jumping

Jumping requires explosive power generation and a strong posterior chain (that's the backside). NFL athletes are tested in the combine on the broad jump and vertical jump because of how telling they are for power generation, and thus, athletic performance.

Gymnasts utilize jumping as an integral part of their training. Basketball players must jump for their sport. For some people, having a weakness in this single skill could result in losing a professional contract worth millions of dollars!

Whether you are an athlete or not, jumping is a skill we all need to train—who knows, it could even save your life someday.

Train your Jumps in as many ways as possible: over, under, on top of, sideways, backwards, long, short, high. Make sure you absorb the shock of your landings by utilizing a squat at the end of each jump (or a roll). You don't want that force to be absorbed by your knees.

43. Train Planks Often

I've heard many coaches or athletes tout planks as their "secret" for getting washboard abs. Meh, diet is the secret.

That said, planks still do amazing things for your abs, obliques, and lower back. I personally love planks for training my lower back (I have anterior pelvic tilt and my lower back is a weakness).

The thing with planks is they are mental. Your results come after your arms start shaking and your mind has told you "enough already" at least 5 times.

44. Work On Your "Rack" Position

Most inexperienced trainees, when they first learn the rack position, have a tendency to keep their elbows back while trying to hold the barbell at the top of the chest. This is incorrect.

A correct rack position has the barbell rested on the "shelf" your shoulders create when you pull them forward and your head back. Your arms should not support the weight at all; your hands are only there to hold the bar in place on your shoulders.

A simple way to test/train the rack position is to put an empty barbell on your shoulders before slowly removing your hands from the barbell and pointing them out in front of you like a zombie. This will show you how a barbell should rest when in the rack position.

To get this form down you must develop the wrist flexibility to be able to hold the barbell in this position (practice). (Picture help: www.agymlife.com/movements)

45. Train Squats! Work Heavy, Light, And Moderate Weighted Squats Every Week

Squats are king. This is what Mark Rippetoe has to say about the squat:

"There is simply no other exercise, and certainly no machine, that provides the level of central nervous activity, improved balance and coordination, skeletal loading and bone density enhancement, muscular stimulation and growth, connective tissue stress and strength, psychological demand and toughness, and overall systemic conditioning than the correctly performed full squat."

Nuff said. Do squats.

(Females take note: Squats form the best parts of your figure.)

46. For Your Weakest Movements, Do This: 3 Sets Of 10 Reps As A Part Of Your Warm-Up And Cool-Down Each Workout

The key to improving movement-based weaknesses is to complete lots and lots (and lots) of reps... but that's not the only thing: you also should train them slow and controlled to develop awareness of your movement. Slow movement allows you to figure out where you suffer from imbalances, flexibility issues, and poor movement patterns.

You can use this technique to improve your weaknesses anytime, not just during your warm-ups. As your weaknesses get stronger, increase the speed and load of reps. Eventually, after you train your weaknesses enough, they'll turn into strengths. That's the goal.

47. Learn From Other Athletes

You never know whom you can learn from. In fact, you can learn something from everyone! We all take a different path to results-land: we all use different tips, tricks and techniques to get there.

Learn from everyone.

Just make sure you take recommendations with a grain of salt, and consider getting a second opinion if it sounds a bit "out there." Then—as with all recommendations—test it out for yourself. If it works for you, great, if not, toss it.

48. Focus On Improving Your Weaknesses

We all hate training our weaknesses. For many of us, this is the reason they are weaknesses in the first place: because we don't train them enough. But if you want to become the best version of yourself possible, you must constantly bring up the levels of your weakest areas in flexibility, endurance, strength, movement, running, rowing, swimming, climbing, gymnastics, and skills related to your sport.

We all like to train what we like to train. This might be because we feel strong doing so or because we have a "love" for certain methods like running or swimming. You have to balance your *favorites* with the all the other parts of your fitness or you'll do your body—and results—a huge disservice.

We all want to be better. Some might want to get better for a sport or specific goal. Others just want to look good naked. No matter the goal, training your weaknesses brings you there faster. You might not always see the connection, but trust me, it's all connected.

Start thinking of your body as one unit. Then aim to make it awesome, bulletproof, strong, well rounded, world-class, and **FIT**. Strive for fitness and everything else will work itself out.

49. Practice Olympic Weightlifting With A Dowel and Empty Barbell

The Olympic lifts—clean, jerk, and snatch—are extremely skill-intensive movements. In fact, these three movements comprise an entire Olympic sport! Like other Olympic sports, athletes train for years to reach competition level. I'm pointing this out to remind you of the importance of taking your time to learn and properly practice these movements.

You should not presume to think you can grab a barbell and start performing heavy Oly lifts. That'll just lead to injury. However, you can grab an empty barbell and start practicing these movements—and move to light weights soon after.

Doing Olympic lifts without proper practice and supervision is a recipe for injury. Obviously, if you are training for the games, I don't need to tell you why you should get better at the Olympic lifts. As with all movement training, the key to progress is lots and lots of reps using light weight followed by slowly, and intelligently, adding load and volume.

The Olympic lifts are an amazing training tool for developing full-body power and speed like none other. If you are new to Olympic weightlifting then I suggest you seek out a local affiliate and find an experienced coach to work with.

50. Listen To Your Body

We all have our own set of genetics. These genetics determine everything relating to your fitness: how flexible you are, how fast you recover and improve, how much muscle you build, where your redline is, what your endurance is for long distances and so on.

When it comes to fitness, we are all different.

You and I cannot train the same way and expect the same results. There is a reason Rich Froning wins the games every year (and it's definitely not his nutrition).

The most important aspect of your training is to LISTEN TO YOUR BODY and respect what it tells you!

My fitness mantra is "test and tweak." This means you listen to your body and adjust volume, weights, nutrition, and lifestyle factors to constantly be searching for the program that brings you the best results. It's an almost never-ending process. You can always find improvement if you are constantly testing and tweaking.

What people don't understand about fitness (and much of life) is just how different we all are, and the role this plays in the results we each get. Too many new, starry-eyed trainees think they can follow Rich Froning's program and magically get similar (or the same) results. Global fitness development isn't a simple linear process (like weightlifting tends to be). There are too many variables to consider. Yet trying to fit everyone into the same box is what many programs, gyms, trainers, and coaches try to do.

For better or worse, your body is your body and you have to find the perfect program for it. Unfortunately, you and I were not born with a manual that tells us what works best for our "model" of human. The only way we figure this out is through lots and lots of training and testing.

You must learn when you can push past your redline and when your body needs a break. You must constantly bring your body to its limit before tapering off so it can heal and adapt. You have to figure out which foods cause you issues, and which you perform best on—the same goes for sleep.

If your nutrition sucks, you shouldn't worry too much about your training other than showing up and doing the work. Remember, nutrition comprises as much as 80% of your body health, composition and performance. Nutrition is fuel; it is the stuff that repairs your body as it adapts to exercise and what it "runs on" during exercise.

Nutrition is the single greatest determining factor in how well your body looks and performs.

If you put unleaded fuel (cheap, processed food) into your body when it really needs rocket fuel (real, whole foods), you will see a lack of results across the board.

No matter what you do: listen to your body. Then use that feedback to make positive changes.

Bonus Tips:

-Don't cherry pick your workouts. The days that your workout makes you want to hide are the days you should NEVER MISS.

-The hardest path is your most direct path to improvement. Make this your default mindset.

-Utilize your coaches before and after class. They love to talk training, food and lifestyle. Ask them questions and then shut up and listen. You will learn a lot.

-Buy a jump rope and size it to you. Never leave it at the gym.

-Don't assume you'll "get big."

Those of you with certain genetics might get bigger, but most of you won't without massive, life-changing effort (and/or drugs). If you decide you do want to get big, make sure you first weigh the pros and cons before making the commitment. With everything you do, you sacrifice something in exchange for something else. If you want to get bigger, you'll have to sacrifice other things like health, time, flexibility, function, money, etc. Make sure it's worth it.

My advice is aim to be fit and proportional. I'll take the lean, ripped, and "fit" look over the "big" look any day. The "get big" trend is dying out. Being bigger won't make you better; it'll just make you bigger. Something to think about.

If you decide to pursue this path you should know that you are fighting your genetics every step of the way. And doing so—one way or another—is going to cause complications in your health.

We all have a genetic predisposition for size. For most of us this ends up being a "lean" and "fit" look that is functional and proportional. Find out what your body type is, accept it, and then work towards making it the best it can be.

Do you think everyone can be the next Arnold? Of course not. He had a one in a billion physique (and mindset).

-To get big you must eat big. Aim for 1-2 grams of protein per pound of bodyweight. Utilize a ton of healthy fat. Get enough carbs from sweet potatoes, yams, white rice, and a hoard of vegetables. Use mass-gainer shakes of the finest ingredients.

-Stay consistent and take a week off every couple months. It will improve your results. Training breaks down your body. Rest builds it up.

-If you want the slim and fit look, you have to lift weights and eat clean. There is no way around it.

-Practice Double-unders every day. DU's are a very skill-intensive exercise: they take lots of practice.

-Don't throw your barbell or equipment. It shows a lack of respect for your gym and the other members that use it every day. Plus, you look like a douche.

-Target "pushing" and "pulling" exercises in your training.

Examples of pushing: press, bench, push-ups,
Examples of pulling: deadlift, pull-up, row

-Swim. Swimming is one of the best low-impact, low-stress and natural movements a human can do to improve his or her fitness. It's so damn good for you. Being a better swimmer can also save your life.

-Work on mobility and keep your joints healthy.
Resource: Kelly Starrett MobilityWod.com

-Don't overtrain. There is too much of a good thing.

-Rest 1-2 minutes between sets. Watch the clock—take your rest intervals seriously.

Warm-up to your heavy sets slowly. Don't just slap 225 pounds on the bar and start squatting. That is a perfect way to hurt yourself.

-Make Kale Chips

These are nutritionally dense, tasty, and super easy to make.

Recipe:
1. Preheat oven to 350
2. Remove leaves from stems
3. Drizzle with oil (I use MCT oil)
4. Bake until edges brown, 10-15 minutes
5. Season with seal salt
6. Enjoy

Eat coconut in many forms. Coconut is a miracle food. Check out the many things you can do with coconut (in addition to eating it). Ways to use: www.agymlife.com/coconut-oil

Play sports and games. Join an adult sports league, go to the park and shoot some hoops, get outside and chase your dog, play beach volleyball, etc. Aim for once a week or at least a few times a month—the more the better.

Sports and play can compliment your fitness like none other. It'll help target weaknesses you might be missing in your training.

Examples of play include:

Running
Jumping
Balancing
Climbing
Swimming
Hand balancing

Places to play:
Parks
Fields
Forest
Jungle
Beach
Mountain
Hill
Trees
Playgrounds
Trails

Sports and games:
Flag football
Dodgeball
Baseball
Kickball
Tennis
Obstacle courses/races
Kayaking
Surfing
Paddle-boarding

Great job... Now get to work!

Thanks for reading. I really, really hope you will take action and start implementing some of these techniques into your program.

Developing habits can be difficult. Keep this in mind when you are trying to implement these new habits in your life. Be prepared to wax and wane during the process... that's to be expected. Just be patient and consistent. Celebrate consistency, not perfection.

Perfection is a fool's errand

Start small: Pick one or two techniques at a time and do them consistently until they "stick." Then add one or two more and repeat the process. Keep building habit upon habit until you end up with the program that is getting you the results you always dreamed of!

This crazy thing we call *health and fitness* is all based on our habits. Keep building them and you will get there. Just keep going no matter what.

If you ever need any help or have any questions, please shoot me an email: ismynamecolin@gmail.com

Yours in Fitness,

-Colin Stuckert

Resources

The following section includes quotes and links from the top experts in the world on all things fitness and training. I owe much of my education to them. You should definitely check them out. Also, there is something you should know about fitness:

There are many ways to skin a cat.

Some coaches produce world-class Olympic athletes using one style while others might use a completely different method and still send their athletes to compete for the gold. Keep that in mind the next time someone tells you this is the "only" or "best" way to train. Always test protocols for yourself. Avoiding buying into any one fitness dogma, and never be closed-minded with your education. *Always be learning.*

Each human body will adapt differently to different forms of training. Some modalities will complement the things you are better at while others might target your weaknesses.

I've said it before and I'll say it again: you must figure it out for yourself. You and you alone have the best *operational manual* for yourself. No one can tell you what your body is telling you. Listen to it.

Kelly Starrett:
http://www.mobilitywod.com/about/kellystarrett/

Author of Becoming a Supple Leopard and founder
MobilityWod.com

Louie Simmons: http://www.westside-barbell.com

Powerlifting legend and Founder/owner of Westside Barbell and author of numerous books and articles

Mark Rippetoe: http://startingstrength.com

Author of Starting Strength

Mark Sisson: http://marksdailyapple.com

My go-to resource for all things ancestral-based health and nutrition. His site is all you need to learn everything you need to know about optimal health and nutrition.

Dave Asprey: http://www.bulletproofexec.com

The Bulletproof Exec and founder of the wildly successful Bulletproof Radio Podcast. His podcast is a must-listen.

Robb Wolf: http://robbwolf.com

My introduction to Paleo eating when I started out some 5 years ago. Robb is a pioneer of the Paleo movement and his podcast is great.

This short list comprises the majority of resources that have contributed to my education on these topics. You should buy their books, subscribe to their podcasts and newsletters, and support them anyway you can.

Tools

Fasting:

Leangains.com
MarksDailyApple.com

Exercise:

5/3/1 Program by Jim Wendler

Nutrition:

Bulletproofexec.com
Robbwolf.com
MarksDailyApple.com

Various Tools I Use:

A Small Crockpot: This thing is AMAZING; consider getting 2 and loading them up each morning
Big Crockpot: great for bigger meals
Victorinox Chef Knives: Cheapest knives that still provide amazing results
Magic Bullet: I use this thing for my Bulletproof Coffee and protein shakes
Aero Press: Preferred way to brew coffee
French Press: 2nd preferred way to brew coffee. Also great for brewing loose tea
Cast-iron skillets: Last a lifetime, get an 8,10 and 12 inch)
Lacrosse ball: For trigger-point release

Food Ingredients:

Bulletproof Coffee
MCT oil
Kerrygold Butter
Himalayan Sea Salt

Supplements:

Ciltep By Natural Stacks
Performance Essentials stack by Natural Stacks
ZMA by Now Foods
Vitamin D by Now Foods
Vitamin C by Now Foods

Books:

GymLifeCook.com: My book on cooking technique. Learn how to cook meals without the use of recipes by learning basic cooking technique you can use over and over.
GymLifeBook.com: My first book on all things fitness and health based on my work at agymlife.com
Tao of Jeet Kune Do: Bruce Lee is my childhood idol. This book is not just about fighting, it's pack-loaded with philosophy.
The Alchemist: International bestseller.
The Four-Hour Body: Tim Ferris fan. Check out his books.
The Richest Man in Babylon: Great book on money.
The Art of Living: The Classical Manual on Virtue, Happiness, and Effectiveness: This book can change your life. It had a role in changing mine.

About The Author

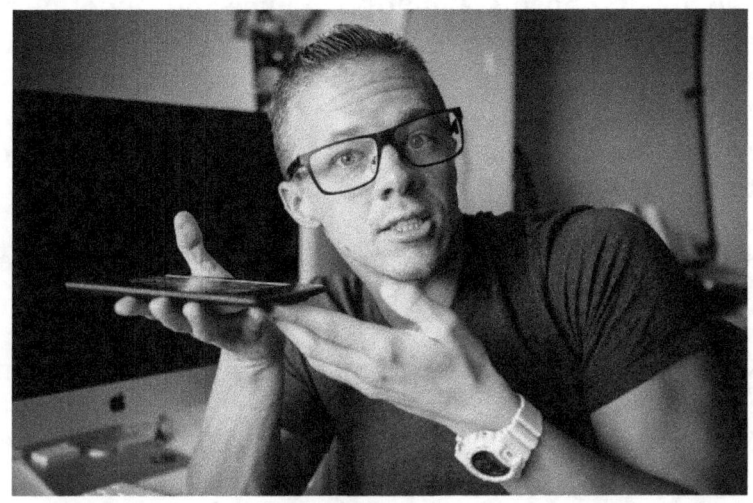

My name is Colin and I'm obsessed with personal development, food and fitness. Like Bruce Lee—my childhood idol—I believe in personal responsibility. What I get in my life is based on me. What you get in yours is based on you. Instead of complaining about the fairness of life and the good luck of others, I'd rather get working and make myself better.

"Time means a lot to me because you see I am also a learner and am often lost in the joy of forever developing."
                    -Bruce Lee

Of course, this isn't the easiest path. It's much easier to sit on the couch and make excuses. It's hard to do work every day... especially when it feels like you aren't moving anywhere... <u>but this is exactly what it takes</u>.

While others will quit after the grind sets in and their motivation wanes, I'll be plowing through (and I hope you will as well). And this is, in my opinion, what separates the winners from the losers, the wheat from the chaff, the cream to the top, the cat from the mouse, and so on.

What I do for a living

I started my first business in 2009: a juice and smoothie bar located inside a large corporate gym (ironic, I know). I started my second business 8 months later a few miles down the road—The Training Box—a group fitness and MMA gym. As I'm writing this, it's been 5 and a half years of learning, blood, sweat and tears, more learning, wasting money, making some back, being sued, spending (we call it "reinvestment" but sometimes I'm not so sure of the difference), plenty of stress, more learning, and now here.

I've worked *really* hard to grow my businesses to be as self-sufficient as possible. Recommend book on the subject: The E-Myth Revisited. Since I've been fortunate enough to attract a great group of people to work in my businesses, I now have the freedom of not having to work "in" my businesses, which allows me the time to pursue other passions (like writing). But it's still a lot of work. In fact, 95% (maybe more) of what it takes to run a business goes on behind "closed doors."

I went to college for a couple years but didn't do well. I stopping going right before speech class credit was due because I was afraid to speak in front of people (which is ironic considering I've had to use this very skill on a daily basis since I started teaching classes at our Box). *But such is life.* I never did well in school and I was always led to believe that I wasn't "smart" or that I would grow up to be a "loser." That's what they convince you of anyway.

When I discovered that you can work hard in your own business to determine your results, I was hooked. To me, personal development and success in business go hand-in-hand. Actually, I can't imagine being that good at business if you aren't good at making yourself better. It's the "always improving" mindset that succeeds. You have to face challenges head on and hustle to overcome them—and learn from the lessons so you are better next time.

Of course, there are many people that work hard, neglect their health, and still get results in certain areas of life. The thing is, I believe these poor souls could get more much greater results—plus all the benefits of being healthy—if they took a health-first approach. Personally, I'm utterly useless if I'm sick or tired. I just curl up in a little ball and my motivation to do anything disappears. This is why, for me, health always comes first. When I feel my best, I perform my best. When I improve myself, I get better at everything else. *This is my fundamental approach to life.*

I've meet many of these not so healthy yet uber-successful people over the years and their situations have always perplexed me. What's the point of having money if you can't enjoy it? Is it really worth working 80 hours a week just so you can watch the numbers in your bank account tick upwards? I don't get it.

If it were me, I would be traveling the world and getting into as much adventure as my success could finance. I would spearfish off the coast of Caribbean islands in a chartered boat, scuba dive in Australia near the great barrier reef, surf in Hawaii, climb mountains, experience new cuisines, meet interesting people from around the world, train with the Shaolin monks, learn urban survival from navy seals, and continually train to become the best version of myself possible and pursue causes that mattered to me. I guess everyone *is* different.

Food and Health

I'm obsessed with food and nutrition. I love to cook and I love to experience the best food I can find. I believe food is the most potent player in the health and longevity of a human being. I eat a Paleo and Primal style diet that consists of some dairy and no grains. I will have a "cheat" meal or two on the weekends, but for the most part I remain gluten-free. If I'm out of town and the occasion calls for it—like in Chicago for deep-dish pizza—I'll have grains. Other than that, I avoid grains because of their inflammatory effects on the body (and so should you).

If there were only one thing you could away from my work it would be **the importance of food.** You have to start eating real food if you want the best results, and/or to enjoy a long and healthy life. There is no way around it—no hack, tip, trick, or shortcut. Maybe when we invent nanotechnology that is able to reverse aging and cure disease, nutrition won't matter. But we don't have that technology, so until we do, food is the epicenter of human existence.

How to eat well:

- Avoid anything processed, refined, synthetic, artificial, etc.
- Cook your food at home so you can control the ingredients.
- Buy the highest-quality food possible.
- Don't eat anything that isn't "real food."

My philosophy

I'm a practicing Stoic. In a nutshell, this means I base my decisions on only what is in my control—like my thoughts, emotions and actions—and I avoid wasting time on things out of my control—like other people, the weather, the past, the future. By taking this pragmatic approach to life, one sees how pointless things like anger, jealously, fear, and worry, actually are. Of course, as with everything, it takes practice. I regularly *catch* myself indulging in negative thoughts even though I've always been an optimist and I'm a consciously practicing Stoic.

I have yet to find a more practical way of living life. This would be my second most potent recommendation for you. Learn about Stoicism and other philosophy. Philosophy has the power to change your life. Here are some resources to help you:

My health and fitness

I average 8-9% body fat year round. This fluctuates up or down depending if I'm traveling or have eating out a lot lately. I lift 3-4 days a week and target each main lift at least once (squat, deadlift, bench, press). I like to use gymnastics as "accessories" to the main lifts. I practice handstands and the basic holds/moves you see break dancers do (and no, I'm not a breaker… maybe one day). I incorporate some full-body functional training like sled work, farmer carries, and tire flips, at least once a week. I need to remind myself to sprint at least once a week. I just started swimming and am kicking myself for not utilizing this amazing form of exercise sooner.

Life

I'm passionate about life and aim to live each day to the fullest. Although this is tough as I often run into the problem of feeling like I'm not doing enough. This is a fault I struggle with. It's the byproduct of being too forward-minded. I tend to forget what *I've already done* and find myself focusing too much on *what I need to do*. I often have to remind myself to take breaks and spend time with friends and family.

I believe that relationships should be a constant pursuit in our lives. They are one of the most important things, if not thee most important. Unfortunately, I feel like so many of us let our relationships suffer when other things start monopolizing our time. And I think it's a grave mistake. Your work, school, project, or whatever should never take precedence over your relationships. Your relationships should always come first. (This is as much a reminder for myself as it is my advice to you.)

My Work

Nowadays, I work with a couple clients in a consulting capacity to help them improve their web presence and marketing. I manage my two businesses and I spend the rest of my time writing, reading and researching topics of interest.

My ultimate dream is to make my full-time income from my writing. Since you are reading this, you have brought me one step closer to that dream. I don't take that lightly.

Thank you so very much.

My other books are available on Amazon (here). I put out a ton of free content on my website AGymLife.com and the corresponding newsletter at GymLifeClub.com. If you want to get all the updates and exclusive list-only content, stop by and subscribe.

If you ever have any questions or need any help, please shoot me an email: ismynamecolin@gmail.com.

I'm here to help anyway I can. At the very least, feel free to share your comments by dropping me a quick note. It's always awesome to get words of encouragement from you guys that help me stay motivated. Amazon reviews also help (I print them out and put them on my wall)!

Yours in Fitness,

-Colin Stuckert

Training Reference Guide
Get this in a PDF guide by going to
www.GymLifeClub.com

Here is an easy-to-remember template for your average training week:

Lift weights and train conditioning three times a week.
Do something longer-distance at least once a week.
Do at least one maintenance session a week.
Get outdoors and do random stuff at least once a week.
Walk every day.

A Hypothetical Training Week:

Monday: Squats followed by a sled-conditioning workout. 15 minutes of skill work at a moderate pace.
Tuesday: Play a pick-up basketball game. A 20-minute walk after dinner. A few sets of push-ups and stretching at home.
Wednesday: Bench press and upper body accessory work. Row 2500m at a slow-medium pace. Yoga for 15 minutes as a cool-down.
Thursday: Walk on the beach. Relax and smell the roses. This is known as a "rest day."
Friday: Active recovery session and skill work for 1.5 hours in the gym. Legs sore from earlier in week so decide to work upper-body gymnastics (handstands, dips, rings). Ride bike for 20-minutes at a medium pace to speed up recovery.
Saturday: Lifting session of deadlift, Olympic weightlifting work, and GHD sit-ups. Beach volleyball, walk on beach, and enjoy a hard-earned cheat meal.
Sunday: Five-mile bike ride at a leisurely pace. Spend two hours prepping food for week. Do 100 push-ups, sit-ups, and squats at home at a slow-medium pace.

The Training Session Format:

1) Body Temp Warm-up: Jog, Row, and move for 5 minutes until you break a sweat.

2) Dynamic Warm-up: Do movement based exercises at slow/light intensity to warm-up and loosen your joints.

3) Strength: Perform one or two main lifts a day to failure. Follow a program or stick with 5 sets of 5 at a weight you can barely complete on your last set.

4) Accessory Exercises: Choose 2-5 complimentary exercises and perform 8-15 reps over 3-5 sets. For example, do pistols (single-leg squats), weighted lunges, and glute-ham raises on your squat days, and do dips, floor presses and clapping push-ups on your chest/shoulder day.

5) Conditioning: Complete 5-25 minutes of high-intensity conditioning work.

6) Cool-down: Stretch, jog, walk, and keep moving for 5 minutes to let your body cool down gradually.

Set Schemes:
10 sets of 2 reps
8 sets of 4 reps
6 sets of 3 reps
5 sets of 5 reps
3 sets of 10
2 sets of 15+
1 set of 21+

WOD types:
AMRAP (as many rounds or reps as possible in X time) 5, 7, 9, 10, 12, 15, 20+ minutes
For Time: 2, 3, 4, 5+ rounds of 2, 3, 4, 5+ exercises for X reps (example= 5 rounds of 10 pull-ups, 10 pushups)
For Time: 100 reps of X
Tabata interval: any exercise or combination of exercises (4 min interval = 20 seconds work, 10 seconds rest until 4 minutes is complete)
10 50m sprints with rest between

In a pinch workouts:
Do a home/travel workout

1 mile run
5x 100m sprints
10x 50m sprints
For time: 100 pushups, 100 sit-ups, 100 air squats
For time: 50 push-ups, 50 air squats
For time: 100 burps (or as many as possible in 7 minutes)

Body Temp warm-up (3-5 minutes of light activity):
Row 500m
Run 500m
5 minutes jump rope
Incline walks
Bike

Dynamic Stretching Warm-up (5-7 minutes of movement-based stretching and moving)(mix these up in various reps and sets):
Squats
Lunges
Arm slaps
Arm circles
Wrist rolls
Neck rolls
Side bends
Runner's lunge
Push-ups
Sit-ups
Jumping jacks

Big Lifts for Strength (choose 1-2 for day):
Back Squat and variants: Front Squat, Overhead Squat, Box Squat
Deadlift and variants: sumo, stiff leg, Romanian,
Press and variants: push press, jerk, split jerk, seated
Bench Press and variants: floor press, DB press, incline, decline
Clean and variants: squat, power
Snatch and variants: squat, power

Common accessory exercises (choose 2-4 per strength exercise above as a compliment):
Squats
Deadlifts
Press
Jerk
Push-ups
Dips
Pull-ups
GHD sit-ups
Back extensions
Good mornings
Clean
Snatches
Kettle bell swings

Conditioning (5-20 minutes of various conditioning modalities):
5 mins - 10 mins - 12 mins - 15 mins - 20 mins - 30 mins - 60 minutes (sometimes)
Strongman
Circuits
Intervals (Tabata)
Swimming
Biking
Hiking
Play a sport

Cool-down (move for 3-5 minutes after workout):
Walking
Stretching
Skill work

Home/Travel WOD workouts requiring no equipment:
-For Time: 10 rounds of: 10 push-ups, 10 sit-ups, 10 squats
-For Time: 50 squats, 50 push-ups, 50 sit-ups
-For Time: 5 rounds of: Run 50m, 10 push-ups

-As many rounds as possible in 10 minutes of: 7 squats, 7 push-ups, 15 sit-ups
-Tabata squats - do as many squats as you can for 20 seconds, rest for 10. Repeat for 4 minutes
-For time: Run 1 mile, 100 Pull-ups, 200 Push-ups, 300 Squats, Run 1 mile
-4x 400M sprints - rest between
-10x 50m Sprint
-Run 1/2 mile 50 air squats – 3 rounds.
-10-9-8-7-6-5-4-3-2-1 sets of sit-ups and a 100 meter sprint between each set.
-Three rounds of: Run 800 meters, 50 Supermans, 50 Sit-ups
-10 push-ups, 10 sit ups, 10 squats – 10x rounds
-200 air squats for time
-3 rounds for time of: Sprint 200m, 25 push-ups
-Run 1 mile, lunging 30 steps every 1 minute.
-Handstand 30-60 second hold on wall and 20 air squats, 5 rounds.
-100 air squats for time
-100 burpees for time
-50 burpees for time
-For time: 4 rounds of: 10 broad jumps, 10 push ups, 10 sit ups
-10 air squats every 1 minute of your 1 mile run
-Run 1 mile for time

The Gym Life List of Usefulness

The Gym Life Essays: Improve Your Life Through Fitness, Food and Mindset: find it on Amazon

This is my first book (recently updated). Each chapter is an individual chapter with topics ranging from improving your fitness, 50 ways to lose weight, how to eat Paleo, and much more.

The Blog: www.aGymLife.com

I write about fitness, lifestyle, mindset, nutrition and health. New articles go up about once a week and I send an exclusive "only to my list" piece every Sunday.

The Gym Life Videos: www.GymLifeVideo.com

I make videos when I can find the time. There are a bunch of 20 Second Recipes videos. Check em out.

The Gym Life Podcast: iTunes

This is my new big project. Make sure you subscribe for all the updates. There are currently 14 episodes up. Feel free to listen and leave a review!

The Gym Life Library of Useful Stuff: http://agymlife.com/better/

This is a collection of bits of content ranging from books I recommend, quotes, tips, tricks, articles, videos, and anything else I find that I think is useful.

Disclaimer:

Consult a doctor before you engage in any exercise program.

The information provided in this book is designed to provide helpful information on the subjects discussed. This book is not meant to be used, nor should it be used, to diagnose or treat any medical condition. For diagnosis or treatment of any medical problem, consult your own physician. The publisher and author are not responsible for any specific health or allergy needs that may require medical supervision and are not liable for any damages or negative consequences from any treatment, action, application or preparation, to any person reading or following the information in this book. References are provided for informational purposes only and do not constitute endorsement of any websites or other sources. Readers should be aware that the websites listed in this book may change.

This book is designed to provide information and motivation to our readers. It is sold with the understanding that the publisher is not engaged to render any type of psychological, legal, or any other kind of professional advice. The content of each article is the sole expression and opinion of its author, and not necessarily that of the publisher. No warranties or guarantees are expressed or implied by the publisher's choice to include any of the content in this volume. Neither the publisher nor the individual author(s) shall be liable for any physical, psychological, emotional, financial, or commercial damages, including, but not limited to, special, incidental, consequential or other damages. Our views and rights are the same: You are responsible for your own choices, actions, and results.